# Stop Hypothyroidism

I0488275

## *Take Control of Your Thyroid & Restore Your Health Naturally*

Christine Weil

© 2014

**All Rights Reserved. No part of this publication may be reproduced in any form or by any means, including scanning, photocopying, or otherwise without prior written permission of the copyright holder.**

Disclaimer and Terms of Use: The Author and Publisher have strived to be as accurate and complete as possible in the creation of this book, notwithstanding the fact that they do not warrant or represent at any time that the contents within are accurate due to the rapidly changing nature of the Internet. While all attempts have been made to verify information provided in this publication, the Author and Publisher assume no responsibility for errors, omissions, or contrary interpretation of the subject matter herein. Any perceived slights of specific persons, peoples, or organizations are unintentional. In practical advice books, like anything else in life, there are no guarantees of income made or health benefits received. This book is not intended for use as a source of medical, legal, business, accounting or financial advice. All readers are advised to seek services of competent professionals in medical, legal, business, accounting, and finance matters.

Printed in the United States of America

# Table of Contents

# Introduction

I want to thank you and congratulate you for purchasing, ***Stop Hypothyroidism: Take Control of Your Thyroid & Restore Your Health Naturally***. You've just made a great decision, in your effort to regain your health. This book contains terrific information and suggestions to treat hypothyroidism, and help you to regain your health and sense of wellbeing.

Do you need that extra cup of coffee or energy drinks to refresh yourself?

Do you feel exhausted, and is your energy sapped all the time?

Do you constantly feel cold?

Do you suffer from unexplained weight gain, constipation, lethargy, and drowsiness, and in general have a low metabolic rate?

If the answer to these questions is a yes, then you may suffer from hypothyroidism or an underactive thyroid gland.

Maybe you are already aware of this fact, and the numerous tests and visits to your doctor seem like a waste of time, as nothing seems to make you feel better. Moreover, the hormone replacement therapy or your thyroid pill may be doing nothing but increasing your discomfort. Do not feel disheartened or anxious if you or your loved one is suffering from this disorder. This book will answer all of your questions with easy, attainable, and effective solutions. Also, these solutions are cost-effective!

5

This book will give you essential information about what hypothyroidism is, what causes it, what worsens your symptoms, and how to treat it and heal your thyroid with lifestyle changes, wholesome nutritious foods and recipes, exercise, and home remedies and holistic healing with homeopathy.

"Life isn't about waiting for the storm to pass .It's about learning to dance in the rain."
— Vivian Greene

Wake up and live your life! Fight your personal storm, equipped with the important and effective tools in this book. This information will help you take control of your thyroid appropriately.

Christine Weil

# What is Hypothyroidism?

The Oxford's Medical Dictionary defines hypothyroidism as, "A condition due to deficient secretion of thyroid." The term hypothyroid is derived from the Greek word "hypo," which means under, and "thyroid" for the thyroid gland.

Hypothyroidism is also known as "underactive thyroid gland." This alternative name comprised of three simple words explains this disorder accurately. Hypothyroidism is an endocrine disorder that results from the inability of your thyroid gland to produce adequate thyroid hormones. Such malfunctions of your thyroid gland, and the resulting low thyroid hormone levels have far-reaching effects on your body. This is because the thyroid gland, through its hormones, regulates your body's metabolism, which is the process of energy production in your body. This important process involves every cell in your body and enables the different organs and glands to work in harmony. Therefore, you may end up feeling fatigued, listless, cold, constipated, and depressed, in addition to gaining weight rapidly.

## Statistics related to hypothyroidism

Women are five to eight times more often afflicted with hypothyroidism than men. It usually occurs in individuals over 50 years of age. However, its incidence in the younger population has also increased in recent years. This is mainly due to the fast-paced, modern life that we live today, full of stress and unhealthy habits. Around 20 million Americans suffer from thyroid diseases. Approximately 60% of these individuals are unaware of their underlying thyroid dysfunctions, as this disorder seldom causes symptoms in the early stages. The American Thyroid Association also estimates that one in every eight women will develop a thyroid malfunction at some point in her lifetime.

The above statistics may seem alarming, but there is still hope. There is no need to be disheartened if you or a loved one are diagnosed with hypothyroidism. This book will equip you with a systematic approach that includes information about nutritious foods and recipes, natural remedies, prescription drugs, and lifestyle changes to heal yourself. If you have been suffering from hypothyroidism for years, and western medicine has done nothing but added to the long list of your health problems, by the time you finish with this book, you will have gained enough knowledge and understanding to take control of your health.

## Normal thyroid functions

To understand hypothyroidism, you need to be familiar with normal thyroid functions and its control mechanisms.

The thyroid is a butterfly-shaped gland located at the front of your neck, a little below the Adams apple. It is a vital component of your endocrine system, along with the pineal gland, the pituitary gland, and hypothalamus in your brain, the pancreas, the testes (males), and the ovaries (females). The endocrine system secretes and regulates the hormones in your body.

Your thyroid secretes a group of hormones known as the thyroid hormones into your blood stream. These hormones include Triiodothyronine or T3, tetraiodothyronine or thyroxine or T4, and calcitonin. The Thyroid Stimulating Hormone, or TSH, secreted by your pituitary gland, makes sure that your thyroid does not produce too little or too much of these hormones.

In addition, iodine absorbed through food is an essential element required for the synthesis of these thyroid hormones. T4 is secreted in relatively higher quantities as compared to T3, and some amount of T4 is converted into active T3 in your blood.

These hormones travel through your blood stream and influence almost every region of your body, including your brain, heart, muscles, and skin. The thyroid gland regulates the production and utilization of energy in your body, as well as normal growth and maturation.

A normal or increased metabolic rate is evidence of a normal thyroid gland that secretes optimal levels of T3 and T4. This simply means:

- An increased or normal body temperature;

- A strong heart beat and a pulse rate between 70-100 beats/minute;

- Quick utilization and absorption of food due to burning of energy resources stored in the muscles and liver;

- A normal body weight;

- Quick reflexes and higher attention span due to activation of the nervous system;

- Promotion of normal growth and brain maturation in children.

Christine Weil

## *Diseased thyroid functions in hypothyroidism*

By now you may have already gauged that hypothyroidism is associated with a slow down in the activity of your thyroid gland. This further leads to reduced secretion of the thyroid hormones T3 and T4. As a result, your blood stream will have lower levels of these crucial hormones.

This results in the pituitary gland working in over-drive to produce more TSH to force the thyroid to increase its hormone secretion, as a defense mechanism of your body. As TSH and iodine are essential for the production of T3 and T4, an abnormally functioning pituitary gland, which is responsible for secreting TSH and monitoring the functions of your thyroid, can also lead to chaotic thyroid functions.

On the other hand, your body does not produce iodine directly but absorbs it through iodine rich foods. Hence, a diet low in this important element can lead to abnormal T3 and T4 levels too. Such sluggish thyroid functions can be present since birth, or may develop during the course of one's lifetime. Low T3 and T4 levels result in a low metabolic rate, which has extensive effects on the overall functions of your body.

Hence, the wide-ranging disease picture of hypothyroidism encompasses sluggishness of reflexes and bodily functions. Very often, hypothyroidism leads to enlargement of the thyroid gland, or goiter, as it's also known. This is due to an increased production of TSH by the pituitary to compensate for the low T3 and T4 hormone levels. The TSH stimulates your thyroid gland and leads to formation of nodules or a bigger thyroid gland.

Western medicine takes into account only the thyroid hormone levels, when it comes to treating hypothyroidism. It completely ignores the diseased thyroid gland in its

enthusiasm to curb the symptoms arising from low T3 and T4 levels.

Although it is important to gain symptomatic relief through these medications, it is also important to heal the underlying cause. Considering the widespread effects of hypothyroidism, a holistic cure that encourages good nutrition and promotes a healthy lifestyle is a natural choice that many people are now embracing.

# What Causes Hypothyroidism?

Your hypothyroid state could be a result of various causative factors. A detailed history of past illnesses, medications, and surgeries helps ascertain the cause in most cases. However, the majority of individuals suffering from hypothyroid do not know what caused it in the first place. Iodine deficiency is the most common cause of hypothyroidism in high altitude areas. On the other hand, Hashimoto's thyroiditis, the autoimmune version of the condition, causes hypothyroidism more frequently in areas with sufficient dietary iodine.

Hypothyroidism is broadly categorized as primary hypothyroidism, in which the cause is within the thyroid gland, and secondary hypothyroidism, when it occurs due to low TSH levels or abnormal activity of the pituitary and hypothalamus.

The possible causes of hypothyroidism are:

- Iodine deficiency: People from developing countries and high altitude areas away from the sea, are more prone to develop iodine deficiency. The addition of iodine to table salt has eliminated this problem in the United States and other developed countries. Seafood, plants grown in iodine-rich soil, and seaweed are the primary sources of dietary iodine.

- Hashimoto's Thyroiditis: This is an autoimmune disorder wherein your immune system produces antibodies that attack and destroy healthy thyroid tissue. Researchers are still not certain as to what causes the immune system to produce these autoantibodies, although some believe viruses, bacteria, or genetic flaws could lead to such a response. Whatever may be the cause, these autoantibodies adversely affect the thyroid gland and its ability to produce hormones.

- Subacute thyroiditis: This is inflammation of the thyroid gland from viral infections such as mumps, Coxsackie, and adenovirus. The thyroid gland is painfully enlarged in thyroiditis, which affects thyroid hormone secretion. There is an initial phase of hyperthyroid (increased thyroid activity) followed by hypothyroidism. If your hypothyroidism is due to subacute thyroiditis, you can undergo complete recovery in four to six months. However, 5 % of subacute thyroiditis cases develop permanent hypothyroidism.

- Thyroid surgery: Thyroidectomy, or removal of all or large portions of the thyroid gland, leads to hypothyroidism, as there is not enough thyroid tissue to produce the required thyroid hormones.

- Radiation: Radiation therapy for cancerous tumors in the neck and head can damage thyroid tissue, resulting in hypothyroidism.

- Treatment for hyperthyroidism: An overactive thyroid gland, or hyperthyroidism, is usually treated with radioactive iodine and anti-thyroid medications. Although these drugs help reduce thyroid hormone levels and stabilize metabolic activity, the downside is that long-term use can cause permanent thyroid damage and hypothyroidism.

- Medications: Certain medicines used in the treatment of cancers, heart diseases, and psychiatric disorders can contribute to the development of

13

hypothyroidism. Lithium used for psychiatric illnesses, amiodarone (cardarone) used for heart problems, interferon alpha, and interleukin-2 are some drugs that can be dangerous for your thyroid.

- Pregnancy: Often, women develop hypothyroidism during or after pregnancy. This may occur because of thyroid inflammation or production of autoantibodies against it. Most women regain their normal thyroid functions after a while, although 20 - 40% of these women remain permanently hypothyroid. Nevertheless, while these hormones remain unstable, careful monitoring is required, as these changes can lead to miscarriages, premature delivery, fetal abnormalities, and preeclampsia or increased blood pressure in the last three months of pregnancy.

- Congenital hypothyroidism: Babies are sometimes born with an underdeveloped or underactive thyroid gland; this condition is recognized as congenital hypothyroidism. Certain congenital birth defects or developmental abnormalities, iodine deficiency in the mother, and autoantibodies can contribute towards this type of hypothyroidism. Babies with hypothyroidism seldom show any visible signs at birth. Such undiagnosed babies can experience severe complications related to mental retardation and stunted growth. Hence, screening for hypothyroidism in babies is now mandatory in most U.S. hospitals.

- Pituitary abnormalities: Certain disorders in the pituitary gland can cause reduced production of TSH. This results in low T3 and T4. Pituitary adenomas or tumors, pituitary surgery, radiation, drugs, sarcoidosis, and infections such as tuberculosis and syphilis can interfere with normal pituitary activity.

- Genetic tendency: If you have a parent, sibling, or relative suffering from this disorder, your genetic make-up is probably to be blamed for your hypothyroidism.

- Changes Your Body Undergoes Due to Hypothyroidism

T3 and T4 travel through your blood stream and help co-ordinate a number of bodily functions. As a result, you may experience various changes in your body related to almost every organ and system.

The symptomatic picture of hypothyroidism is extensive as it has a negative impact on your metabolism. In fact, because of this multiple organ involvement, you may even misunderstand a few hypothyroid symptoms for something else.

Hypothyroid has an insidious onset and develops slowly over a period of time, with the expression of subtle symptoms in the beginning. Because of this reason, most people are not even aware that they could be suffering from it. Many people also ignore the mild signs of hypothyroidism in the initial stages, mistakenly attributing them to some other milder illnesses. As a result, an alarming 60% of hypothyroid individuals go undiagnosed.

Listen to what your body tries to tell you, pay attention to every normal or abnormal sensation you experience, as symptoms are the language your body uses to speak to you.

## *Signs and Symptoms of Hypothyroidism*

Your body could be going through few or all of the following changes because of sluggish metabolic activities.

### Thyroid:

- A mild to moderate enlargement of the thyroid gland may be present

- Sometimes this enlargement is visible to the naked eye medically known as goiter

### Gastrointestinal or digestive tract changes

- Decreased appetite
- Constipation due to sluggish bowel movements
- Unexplained weight gain
- Rarely in severe or untreated cases of hypothyroidism, there may be fluid collection in the abdomen

### Heart affections

- Bradycardia or a decreased heart rate below 60 beats/minute
- Increased blood pressure
- Angina or occasional episodes of chest pain or discomfort

- Severe or untreated hypothyroid can also lead to fluid collection around your heart and lungs, and cardiac failure

## Nerve and muscle changes:

- Aches and pains
- Muscle stiffness and cramps
- Swollen and painful joints
- Delayed or sluggish reflexes
- Carpel tunnel syndrome that occurs due to compression of the median nerve at the wrist can be an expression of hypothyroidism too. If you are experiencing pain and numbness along your thumb, index, middle, and some part of your ring finger, you probably have carpel tunnel syndrome.
- Poor hearing due to fluid collection in the middle ear

## Psychological changes

- Lack of concentration and weak memory
- A slow thought process
- Depression and psychosis in severe cases

## Skin changes

- A puffy face
- Dryness of hair and skin
- Increased hair fall that may cause balding.
- Vitiligo or pinkish white patches on skin are also seen in some hypothyroid individuals.
- Swelling of skin around hands, feet, and eyelids

## Reproductive changes:

- Irregular periods and/or heavier menstrual flow
- Decreased sex drive
- Infertility and impotence

## General changes

- Fatigue or increased tiredness
- Shortness of breath
- Excessive drowsiness
- Intolerance or increased sensitivity to cold
- Hoarseness of voice
- Anemia or low hemoglobin levels

As you can see, hypothyroidism shows itself through diverse signs and symptoms.

You may or may not experience all of these symptoms. However, the general changes in metabolism and symptoms are usually common to every hypothyroid individual.

Such sensations and symptoms can be quite frustrating to deal with, especially when at work, during an important meeting, or while you are out shopping or enjoying a movie or an outing.

Not everyone finds complete relief with conventional medicines. Although your conventional medicines are important to avoid complications arising from hypothyroidism, you also require additional props to find complete relief. You can certainly gain the good health and relief you are looking for through wholesome foods, healthy habits, lifestyle changes, and natural alternative therapies mentioned here.

# Monitoring Your Hypothyroid Status

Hypothyroidism is fairly easy to monitor. Your doctor probably orders blood tests every 6 - 12 months to know if your thyroid hormones are stable. This is a good practice, as it will help you understand your position on the road to recovery. So, always stay on schedule when it comes to keeping a check on your thyroid hormone levels.

In addition to the thyroid profile, you may also require a few more tests to make sure that your heart, kidneys, and other organs are in order. These supplementary tests help keep an eye on the progress of hypothyroidism, in addition to examining the possibility of related complications.

Learning to interpret your blood investigation reports and scans is beneficial. Doing so will not only give you enough information about your thyroid gland and body, but it will also save you from unnecessary worrying while you wait to consult your doctor.

## *Blood Tests*

### Thyroid function tests

Thyroid function tests, as suggested by the name, check your thyroid functions by measuring the different hormones and enzymes in your blood stream.

The T3, T4, and TSH levels in your blood are the most important and commonly acknowledged parameters for this purpose. There are two ways to measure T3 and T4 hormones in your blood.

The old method, which is more widely used, measures the T3 and T4 bound partially or completely to the carrier proteins. These carrier proteins transport the hormones through your blood to areas where they are considered necessary.

On the other hand, the newer method, which has gained popularity recently, measures free or unbound T3 and T4 molecules in your blood stream. These free hormone molecules, are actually believed to be responsible in bringing about the biological actions credited to them.

Hence, testing free T3 and T4 gives a more accurate account of your thyroid functions. Another drawback to the old method is that the number of protein carriers often changes in certain medical conditions such as pregnancy, which may result in an inaccurate account of the thyroid hormone levels.

TSH levels are routinely measured to screen thyroid disorders, especially in older people, pregnant women, or women trying to conceive, and infants, as these are high-risk groups of hypothyroidism.

If the TSH levels turn out to be abnormal, then further tests to determine T3 and T4 levels are undertaken to check for hypothyroidism.

| Test name | Normal range | Changes due to hypothyroidism | Preparations before the test |
|---|---|---|---|
| **Serum T3** | 80-180 ng/dl | Low T3 (below 80 ng/dl) | 8-12 hours fasting |
| **Serum T4** | 4.6-12 ug/dl | Low T4 (below 4.6 ug/dl) | 8-12 hours fasting |

| Serum TSH | 0.5-6 uU/ml | High TSH (above 6uU/ml) | 8-12 hours fasting |
|---|---|---|---|
| Free T3 | 230-619 pg/dl | Low free T3 (below 230 pg/dl) | No fasting required |
| Free T4 | 0.7-1.9 ng/dl | Low free T4 (below 0.7 ng/dl) | No fasting required |

***Some variations do occur in these test results, so in case you are suffering from subclinical hypothyroidism, your thyroid hormones or T3 and T4 levels may be within the normal limits, but you will have a substantially raised TSH.

***In rare cases, where hypothyroidism occurs due to pituitary gland failure or abnormalities, there will be low T3 and T4 levels along with a low TSH level, as the pituitary is unable to function normally and produce enough TSH to stimulate the thyroid gland, subsequently lowering T3 and T4 too.

## Lipid profile

The lipid profile measures the levels of different cholesterols and triglycerides in your blood stream. Generally, hypothyroidism and the associated slow metabolism, cause an increase in the serum cholesterol and triglyceride levels.

Cholesterol and triglycerides are the fat and oil content in your blood, which collect along the walls of your blood vessels and my lead to blockages in the long run. This test requires a 12 - 14 hour fasting prior to collection of blood.

The normal lipid profile values of importance are listed below.

| Test | Normal values | Changes due to hypothyroidism |
|---|---|---|
| Total cholesterol | 100-200 mg/dl | High Total Cholesterol (above 200 mg/dl) |
| LDL | Less than 110 mg/dl | High LDL (above 110 mg/dl) |
| HDL | More than 40 mg/dl | - |
| Triglycerides | Less than 150 mg/dl | High triglycerides (above 150 mg/dl) |

***HDL or high-density lipoprotein is more commonly know as good cholesterol, since it has the ability to dissolve fat and oil deposits in your blood vessels. LDL or low density lipoprotein, commonly known as bad cholesterol, is bad for your heart and general health due to its tendency to form deposits.

**Serum sodium levels**

Sodium, Na, or natrum is an element present in your body. It is mainly required for nerve and muscle functions. You may have low sodium levels in your blood stream due to hypothyroidism. Normally, serum sodium values should be between 135-145 mEq/L.

## Complete blood count or CBC

Hypothyroidism is often associated with anemia or low hemoglobin levels in your blood. Your CBC will show low hemoglobin levels if you have anemia. A Hb below 12 mg/dl in women and 14 mg/dl in men is classified as anemia.

## *Scans and Radiograms*

Your doctor will not order these scans and X-rays very often. The commonly performed scans for hypothyroid are electrocardiogram or EKG, chest X-rays or radiograms, thyroid scans, and thyroid ultrasonography. The EKG and chest radiograms usually monitor complications or the effects of hypothyroidism on your heart.

Thyroid scans check thyroid functions, and thyroid USGs help detect anatomical abnormalities such as thyroid enlargement, nodules, and thyroid cancer. If you have hypothyroidism, your EKG will perhaps show bradycardia or a slow pulse rate, low voltage QRS complexes, and ST-T wave abnormalities. In addition, your chest X-ray may show an enlarged heart shadow.

## *The Medical community's outlook towards thyroid testing*

Conventional medicine is extremely dependant on the above tests and diagnostic criteria. However, due to this inflexible attitude towards the diagnosis of hypothyroidism, the medical community often misses diagnosing it or totally misdiagnoses it.

Very often, people show a symptomatic picture of hypothyroidism, but their serum T3 and T4 levels are within the normal limits, and hence do not correlate with this symptomatic picture. Western medicine sometimes sends these patients away with antidepressants or antipsychotics, when what these people actually need are hypothyroid medications. You can have normal thyroid hormones but a raised TSH as seen in subclinical hypothyroid, or you could have normal T3, T4, and TSH levels, but with further tests that may show the presence of thyroid autoantibodies in your blood, leading to a diagnosis of hypothyroidism.

Hypothyroidism is almost 20 times more frequent than hyperthyroidism, and it can go undiagnosed if we stick to the diagnostic criteria set by western medicine. People in the initial stage of hypothyroidism, when the disease is very mild, may show normal TSH values, although they feel tired, cold, sluggish, have trouble concentrating, and gain weight quickly.

Western medicine will surely miss diagnosing such people. Indeed, recent research has lead to a debate amongst the medical community and endocrinologists in particular to reduce the upper limit of the TSH normal range from 6 uU/ml to as low as 3 uU/ml.

In addition, using the old method of measuring the hormones bound to carrier proteins has its drawbacks too. At times, the quest for scientific proof through investigations and diagnostic data can handicap the medical fraternity leading to increased dose adjustments and mix-ups.

It is important to keep in mind that these tests are only props to help you as you heal, and not something you base your decisions on. Often, with lifestyle changes, natural medicines, and alternate therapies you may feel better, but there may be an absence of significant changes in your test results.

This does not mean you discontinue your healing methods because you are not getting better.

You *are* getting better!

A relief in your symptoms is the first sign of improvement and the much-desired test results will follow soon enough. A meticulous and personal approach centered towards complete cure and symptomatic relief is what you require to heal your hypothyroidism.

# Conventional Treatment of Hypothyroidism

The conventional treatment for hypothyroidism is to replace the deficient thyroid hormones in your bloodstream. The criteria to begin with hormone replacement therapy are the presence of hypothyroid symptoms and a confirmed thyroxine or T3 and T4 deficiency. Most people with hypothyroidism respond well to synthetic hormone preparations, but they have to be continued lifelong.

A purely synthetic, laboratory-prepared form of hormone levothyroxine or T4 is widely available as Levothroid and Synthroid, for use in the treatment of hypothyroidism.

A synthetic form of T3 Liothyronine Sodium is also available as Cytomel. However, levothyroxine is the preferred choice of treatment because it is more stable and a single daily dose is sufficient, whereas synthetic T3 is short-acting and requires multiple daily doses. Desiccated thyroid tablets prepared from animal thyroid glands were used previously, but after the entry of synthetic Levothyroxine, these tablets are no longer used in conventional treatments.

Levothyroxine is administered orally in an average dose of 1.6 mcg/kg body weight per day. Typically, a dose of 50 mcg daily for three weeks, followed by 100 mcg daily for three weeks, followed by a maintenance dose of 150 mcg daily is customary practice.

In the elderly and people with heart problems, thyroxine is initiated in a lower dose of 25 mcg daily. This gradual increase in dosage helps your heart and body to adjust to the metabolic changes. The thyroxine dose is adjusted so that the serum TSH levels remain below 3 mU/L.

Always take your thyroxine pills half an hour before breakfast. Also, avoid eating calcium-rich foods and soy a few hours before and after taking these pills, as these food items can inhibit the action of thyroxine.

These medicines can be potentially dangerous when taken improperly or in the wrong dosage. Hence, do not stop your medicines or change your dosage without consulting your doctor. It is also mandatory to monitor the free T4 and TSH levels in your blood 4 - 6 weeks after beginning treatment, or after a change in your thyroxine dose.

The drawbacks of hormone replacement therapy are many. It causes various side effects, and not everyone responds positively to this therapy. Besides, most people continue to experience the distressing symptoms of hypothyroidism regardless of these pills.

Neither does this therapy heal your thyroid or the underlying cause of your hypothyroidism. All it does is replace your hormones.

### Side effects of hormone replacement therapy

Conventional medicine can cause a number of side effects. What's worse is that your doctor may not even tell you about them.

- Excess thyroxine usually leads to insomnia, increased appetite, palpitations in the chest, and shaking or tremors.

- Thyroxine also causes calcium loss from your bones making them weak, and increasing your chances of osteoporosis.

- It also causes or worsens chest pain in people with heart problems. An excess dose of thyroxine also increases the risk of heart attacks in these patients.

## Limitations of thyroxine replacement therapy

- If you are among the lucky few, you may respond to the thyroid pills within one to two weeks, with substantial relief from the symptoms. However, most people take two to three months to feel better with thyroxine.

- It is not always easy to identify the exact suitable dosage of thyroxine. Most people have to undergo numerous tests and dosage adjustments to know what suits them best.

- Other medicines such as antacids, calcium supplements, iron supplements, cholestramine effective in lowering blood cholesterol levels, and seizure medicines interfere with the action of thyroxine, hence they cannot be taken together.

- Patients with subclinical hypothyroidism do not respond to this treatment as they have normal T3 and T4 levels. Thyroxine only helps reduce the risk of heart diseases in these people.

- Stopping this treatment will bring back all of your symptoms and hence it has to be continued lifelong.

Taking in all of this information can be quite overwhelming. You may even feel helpless at times as you deal with hypothyroidism. Nevertheless, there is a simple solution to your predicament. A healthy lifestyle with an emphasis on nutritious foods, adequate physical activity, and alternate therapies in addition to thyroxine, is the answer to many of your question about hypothyroidism.

# Learn to Balance Your Hypothyroid Naturally

Now that you have a better understanding of hypothyroidism and its effects on your body, we can focus on the most important aspect, which is taking control of your thyroid and healing yourself naturally. The good news is that these methods are much simpler and certainly more effective in comparison to conventional medicine.

## *A Healthy lifestyle*

Taking steps towards a healthy lifestyle may look difficult, but this process is simpler than you think. You can start with baby steps in the beginning. There is no hurry, and this is not a race. However, if you begin taking these positive steps, you will gain better control of your life and heal yourself in no time. Go slowly but steadily, and you will win against your hypothyroidism. Incorporate the following guidelines to live a healthy lifestyle and heal your thyroid.

### Faulty habits and addictions

Unhealthy habits including smoking, alcohol abuse, and the use of recreational drugs can have tremendously harmful effects on your health and thyroid. If you have any such habits, consider discontinuing them. Start taking positive steps towards ridding yourself of addictions, and reclaim your health. If required, do not shy away from taking professional help to get rid of these injurious habits.

**Smoking:** Cigarette or tobacco smoking can produce a notably negative impact on your thyroid functions. A number of studies conducted through the 1980s and 90s confirm that Thiocyanate and Nicotine present in cigarette smoke interfere with thyroid functions. These chemicals can reduce the ability of your thyroid to take in iodine, subsequently hindering the production of thyroid hormones.

As a result, smoking will worsen your symptoms and make your metabolism even more sluggish. Smoking can also increase the amount of TSH in your bloodstream. Hence, if you have subclinical hypothyroidism, it is all the more important for you to stop.

## *Tips to stop smoking*

Nicotine patches and gums, easily available in stores, can help you break this habit. The more recent electric cigarettes available for this purpose also work effectively. Speak to your loved ones so they can support and help you with the process of de-addiction. Reach out for professional help if your personal steps aren't successful.

**Alcohol:** Alcohol stands third among the risk factors for various diseases and disabilities. It is known to cause 60 diseases and contribute to another 200.

Chronic alcohol use can produce toxic effects on your thyroid cells, and a decrease in your thyroid hormones. It also blunts the effects of TSH, further decreasing your thyroid hormone levels. Almost 50.1% of the American population drinks alcohol more often than recommended. Continuing with your alcohol consumption will even nullify all the other positive steps you may take towards healing yourself. Limit your consumption to just one drink or less a day.

## *Tips to limit your alcohol intake*

If you are a regular drinker or are addicted to alcohol, reduce your alcohol intake gradually. Try to indulge in positive activities or hobbies to distract, and keep yourself busy. Ask your loved ones to help and encourage you in your endeavor. Chronic drinkers generally experience withdrawal symptoms such as tremors. Consult your doctor should you experience anything more severe. Seek professional help when required.

**Recreational drugs:** Most Recreational drugs such as cocaine, heroin, marijuana, and amphetamines lead to autoimmune disorders. Cocaine in particular can cause autoimmune disorders of the thyroid such as Hashimoto's thyroiditis. Do not try to de-addict yourself if you use any such drugs, but seek professional help promptly for de-addiction.

# Healthy sleep habits

Sleeping for eight to 10 hours daily is important for general well-being and good health. Good quality and adequate sleep will rejuvenate and refresh you.

The problem with hypothyroidism though, is not lack of sleep but too much sleep. You may feel sleepy and listless very often. Undisturbed and sufficient sleep at the right time can help you counter unnecessary drowsiness. Sleeping well will keep you full of zip, and help you go through your day with energy and enthusiasm.

**Here are some tips for a healthy sleep schedule**

- Sleep for 8-10 hours daily.

- How and when you sleep is important too. If you sleep inadequately or fitfully at night, your chances of feeling drowsy and lethargic through the day are higher.

- Go to bed and wake up at a fixed time everyday. Setting up this sleep-wake schedule may be a little tedious in the beginning but it will get easier as your body adjusts to these changes, and you will start waking up refreshed in the mornings.

- Avoid sleeping or working late. Do not watch television or use your computer, laptop, or iPad late into the night.

- Afternoon naps or siestas are a common trend in many cultures. They are an excellent way to tackle daytime drowsiness and keep you refreshed. Sleeping for 30 minutes to one hour in the early afternoons is a good habit, especially when you have hypothyroidism. Plan your daily routine so that you have time for a quick nap. Naps make up for all the energy loss during the first half of your day, which is usually the busiest time. So, have your power nap without feeling guilty, because it is good for you.

- Melatonin, a hormone secreted by your brain is responsible for inducing and regulating normal sleep. Loss of light normally triggers its production. Hence, if your house or office space is dark during the daytime, increasing your exposure to natural light will help reduce daytime drowsiness. Open the curtains, blinds, and windows in your home and office. Let the sunlight come in. Keep your room well ventilated and well lit. Move your desk closer to the window if possible.

- Avoid having stimulants such as coffee, tea, and caffeinated energy drinks to keep yourself awake. Although these may help keep you awake initially, prolonged use and too much caffeine in your body has an opposite effect and can worsen your drowsiness.

**Some effective sleep promoting techniques to help you sleep better**

- Massage your head with sesame, brahmi, or coconut oil an hour before your bedtime.

- Soothe yourself with a warm bath, and keep the atmosphere in your room cool and dark before your bedtime, so that you fall asleep quickly.

- Having a glass of warm milk, with a pinch of nutmeg powder and a teaspoonful of honey, or a banana, half an hour before your bedtime should help you sleep peacefully through the night.

- Conversely, avoid having bananas or nutmeg during the day as they can increase your drowsiness.

## Stress management

Your exposure to mental and emotional stress can worsen your symptoms. It also causes your hormones to go berserk.

Many doctors and researchers believe that stress can negatively affect your thyroid, as stress leads to increased production of the corticosteroid hormone cortisol. Too much cortisol in your body can interfere with the production of thyroid hormones. A study published in the journal "Thyroid" in 2004 states that stress can also cause thyroid autoimmunity and Hashimoto's disease.

Our lives today overflow with stress thanks to the competitive and fast-paced world in which we live. You may have to face undue stress at home and work. Trying to be a super-parent, attending to your children's needs, sticking to deadlines at work, driving through traffic, shopping, and a number of your daily chores can make your stress levels go out of control. Stress also makes a lot of people turn to injurious habits such as smoking, alcohol, and recreational drugs, which are especially harmful if you have hypothyroidism or a genetic tendency for the same.

Learning to minimize your stress is important for good health. Always be optimistic, and put yourself right at the top in your list of priorities. Set realistic goals for yourself, and do not overdo or over-burden yourself with too many changes or new additions to your routine while you pursue good health. Each step you take, however slow it may be, will still get you closer to health and healing your thyroid.

The speed does not matter as long as you do not stray.

### Tips to de-stress

Meditation and yoga can help reduce your stress levels considerably. Another stress-buster is exercise. A daily one-hour workout session can significantly reduce your stress, as exercise makes your brain release endorphins or feel-good hormones. Regular eight to 10 hours of sleep is also essential to de-stress.

### Weight management

When you have hypothyroidism, your metabolism is too slow to process your food properly. As a result, you may gain weight too quickly in spite of a low appetite. You will also find it a little more difficult to shed those extra pounds.

Hypothyroidism can increase your weight by up to 20 pounds. Any weight gain above 20 pounds is usually due to lethargy and lack of physical activity associated with an underactive thyroid.
Always remember that you can lose weight even with hypothyroidism, although the process of weight loss maybe

slower. Don't feel discouraged if your weight loss methods haven't paid off yet.

You will lose weight gradually, with a healthy lifestyle, exercise, and wholesome nutritious foods. Also, avoid overly enthusiastic measures to reach your goal faster such as crash diets and vigorous workouts. They can aggravate your hypothyroidism, and damage your health.

Ideally, your body mass index or BMI should be within 20 to 27. A BMI above 27 - 30 is categorized obese. Keeping your body weight within the BMI of 20 - 27 is necessary in treating hypothyroidism, as weight gain can aggravate the symptoms of hypothyroid and increase your risk of heart diseases.

**Remember the following guidelines while you try to shed those extra pounds.**

- Maintain your BMI below 27.

- Do not diet or stay hungry to lose weight. Crash diets will do nothing but harm your health and metabolism. Eat your meals on time, and avoid skipping them.

- Many herbal remedies for weight loss are available online and in health food stores today. Not all of them work. Avoid such short cuts to lose weight. Some of them may work, but most of them can affect your thyroid gland and hormones adversely. Check the labels and research their ingredients thoroughly before you use them.

- Have a healthy, balanced diet that includes all essential nutrients and wholesome foods.

- Avoid eating processed foods and junk foods. These food items contain added sugars, artificial chemicals, and preservatives. These chemicals can worsen your hypothyroidism and increase weight gain.

- Avoid calorie-rich foods, and fried or oily food items. Such foods promote weight gain.

- Avoid refined carbohydrates and have more proteins in your diet.

## Healthy diet and detoxification techniques

What you eat, how you cook your food, and where you buy your food are all important parameters in the process of healing your body and thyroid. When it comes to taking control of your hypothyroidism and stabilizing your thyroid hormones, it is essential to watch what enters your body through food, especially since weight loss is one of the important goals in treating hypothyroidism.

### Healthy dietary measures for hypothyroidism

A few simple and cost-effective measures towards the correction of your dietary habits can greatly reduce your symptoms. These steps can also improve your thyroid function tests by improving the activity of your thyroid gland. Correct your dietary habits by avoiding faulty eating habits and unhealthy foods.

- *Go organic:* Always buy your food from organic food stores and farmers markets. Look for such stores in your area instead of visiting supermarkets that stock processed and mass-produced food items. Organic foods are produced in natural environments, without the use of artificial hormones, antibiotics, and chemicals such as coloring agents and preservatives. Organically grown produce also has minimum or no pesticides and insecticides. This will considerably minimize your exposure to environmental toxins. Organic food is also healthier and contains essential nutrients in natural forms and quantities.

- *Read labels and nutrition facts:* When you shop for food and groceries, make a habit of reading food labels. Check the nutritional facts to understand the amount of nutrients and calories in the food you are buying. This will help you make correct and informed decisions based on the nutritional value of each product. Checking these labels will also help you stick to your weight loss or maintenance diets more easily.

- *Avoid goitrogenic foods:* Some food types known as goitrogens have anti-thyroid properties and tend to lower your thyroid functions. Soya beans and soy products, millet, cabbage, broccoli, turnips, Brussels sprouts, radishes, asparagus, mustard, peanuts, and pine nuts have goitrogenic effects and should be avoided when you have hypothyroidism. Especially avoid eating these vegetables raw. You can have them occasionally after cooking, as cooking reduces their goitrogenic properties.

- *Avoid processed foods, fast foods, and junk foods:* These food items are high in unwanted calories, artificial sugars, preservatives, added flavors and chemicals. They tend to reduce the nutritional value of your food and promote weight gain. They also increase your toxic load, resulting in a slower metabolic rate. Jams, marmalade, pickles, commercial salad dressings and mayonnaise, and Maple syrup are some food types to avoid.

- *Avoid grains containing gluten:* Barley, rye, semolina, spelt, wheat, and bulgar, are gluten-rich grains. They should be avoided too, as they can lower your thyroid functions.

- *Avoid sugars and refined carbohydrates:* Such food items and drinks are harmful, as they cause blood sugar imbalances and adrenal stress, which in turn lowers your thyroid functions, in addition to promoting unhealthy weight gain. Hence, avoid overly sweet foods, candies, sweetmeats, ice creams, pastries, cakes, cup cakes, popsicles, and bakery products when you have hypothyroidism.

- *Avoid saturated fats and cholesterol rich food items* Hypothyroidism can increase your risk of heart diseases by increasing the tendency of fats to deposit along your blood vessel walls. You may also have high levels of cholesterol and triglycerides in your blood. Hence, is beneficial to avoid fatty, oily, and fried foods. Use coconut oil or olive oil for cooking, as they contain good fats and help reduce cholesterol. Your heart and cholesterol levels may also benefit from having a tablespoon of flaxseeds and two to three almonds daily.

- *Healthy calorie options:* The calories in your diet provide your body with energy. However, it is important that you do not exceed your daily calorie requirement. Your daily calorie intake depends on your weight, height, and physical activity. Ideally, non-overweight women require 2000 calories/day, while non-overweight men require 2600 calories daily. These values may vary based on your lifestyle and level of physical activity. If you are obese or on a weight loss regimen you need to cut down your daily calorie intake by five to 10%. Nuts and seeds, such as macadamia nuts, pecan nuts, walnuts, almonds, sunflower seeds, sesame seeds, flaxseeds, peanut butter, cheese, and dark chocolate are healthy dietary options with high calorific value.

- *Eat more iodine-rich foods:* Your diet is the sole source of iodine for your body, hence you should eat more iodine rich foods such as seafood, seaweeds, kelp, Swiss chard, kombu, minced beef, eggs, sesame seed butter, onions, artichokes, garlic, and vegetables grown in iodine-rich soil. Make sure you buy only iodized salt. Also, do not overdo this as excess iodine can worsen your hypothyroidism

- *Eat more selenium-rich foods:* Brazil nuts, onions, tomatoes, and tuna are some good sources of selenium.

- *Eat more plant and animal proteins:* Proteins are essential in weight loss and muscle building and toning. Hence, it is beneficial to include a plant or animal protein in every meal. Pulses, legumes, beans, sprouts, soya, tofu, eggs, skinless chicken, lean meat, and fresh or frozen fish are rich sources of dietary protein.

- *Have more fruits, vegetables, and whole grains:* Eat more fruits and vegetables, as they are rich sources of essential vitamins, minerals, and micronutrients. Avocados, apples, and pears are good sources of vitamins and antioxidants. Have whole grains such as whole wheat, brown rice, whole wheat brown breads, wheat germ, and barley.

- ***Drink lots of water:*** Hydrate yourself with at least one to two quarts of water daily. This will tackle dehydration and boost your metabolism. This will also relieve constipation.

- *Have more dietary fiber:* Make sure you have 10 - 25g of dietary fiber daily. It is essential to relieve constipation due to hypothyroidism, and remove toxins from your body. Green leafy vegetables, spinach, fenugreek, squash, mushrooms, oats, kidney beans, and berries such as, blackberries, strawberries, gooseberries, raspberries, and cranberries are some sources of dietary fiber. Dried prunes are also rich in dietary fiber and help relieve constipation.

- ***Have more calcium-rich foods:*** Thyroxine therapy usually reduces the calcium in your bones. To counter these effects have a glass of low fat milk, yoghurt, or buttermilk daily. However, make sure you do not have calcium-rich food or supplements along with your thyroid pill.

**Healthy detox habits**

Detoxification techniques and diets have gained a lot of popularity recently. You may have heard about these diets previously and maybe even practiced a few of them previously, but do you know what they really are?

Certain environmental pollutants including poisonous fumes, pesticides such as dioxins, cigarette smoke, artificial food additives, food coloring agents and preservatives, and drugs are known to interfere with the functions of the thyroid gland.

These environmental toxins can inhibit the production of the thyroid hormones by affecting the iodine uptake by your thyroid gland, and worsen your symptoms. Most of these toxins enter your blood stream through the food that you eat. Your body flushes out these toxins naturally when they are in small quantities, but they can be harmful in large quantities.

Toxins generally enter your body and accumulate to dangerous proportions, as the speed at which they enter your body is usually quicker than the speed at which they are eliminated by your body.

It is not very difficult to eliminate these toxins from your body. You can limit your exposure to these harmful substances very easily. Reducing the inflow of toxins through healthy detox enables your body to eliminate the accumulated toxins. In my opinion following three basic rules can help you detox, without much of the detox drama available on the internet these days.

1.  Eat only organic produce as much as possible. Organic food items usually come with a green USDA certified organic seal. Check for this seal on food labels when you go grocery shopping.

2.  Use organic and natural household and personal hygiene products such as hair-care products, shampoos, and detergents.

3. Use home remedies and homeopathy medicines or herbs for common illnesses, instead of popping pills at the drop of a hat.

A lot of the detox diets available today advise extreme measures and crash dieting. In my experience, such programs cause more pain than gain. Hence, avoid jumping on this bandwagon blindly, especially when you have hypothyroidism.

They will do nothing but worsen your condition. You can follow some simple measures to detox yourself. However, remember that detoxification of your system is like spring-cleaning your house. After a while, just as the cobwebs and dust starts coming back, so will your toxins. Hence, repeat such steps weekly or monthly.

**Here is how you can detox with hypothyroidism.**

- Fix three to seven days every month for your detox program.

- Eat fruits and vegetables on these days. Try to have them raw.

- You can have small portions of skinless organic chicken or fish too.
- Eat only steamed or boiled food. Avoid shallow fried or deep fried food and oil.

- Have more salads and soups. You can use fresh parsley and cilantro to season these.

- Avoid seasoning your food with spices.

- Drink loads of water and fresh fruit juices to flush out the toxins from your body.

- Make sure you have healthy and nutritious foods.

- Do not starve your self or go on a total liquid diet as these steps can damage your metabolism.

**Some wholesome recipes for hypothyroidism and detox**

### *Mushrooms and Leek Stir-Fry*

This is a great recipe for people with hypothyroidism. It is a nutritious combination of proteins and vitamins. Additionally, mushrooms have cholesterol-lowering properties, which is an added benefit when you have hypothyroidism.

Ingredients:

3 cups washed and sliced oyster mushrooms

1 cup sprouted beans

1 thinly sliced onion

1 leeks washed and sliced to form rings

3 cloves of crushed garlic and a small piece of crushed ginger

1 carrot washed and sliced

1 tsp cumin seeds

5 oz of rice noodles

½ tsp chili powder

2 tbsp vinegar

1 tbsp coconut or olive oil

Preparation:

1. Boil the rice noodles and keep them aside in cold water.

2. Now add the oil the pan.

3. Add the cumin seeds, ginger garlic paste, and onions and cook for 3 minutes.

4. Add the leeks and let them cook until they turn brown.

5. Now throw in the mushrooms, carrots and beans, and cook until the mushrooms are cooked.

6. Add the chili powder and vinegar as per your taste requirement.

7. Add the noodles and let everything cook together for 3 minutes.

8. Have this warm for lunch or dinner.

## Zucchini and Salmon Salad

This is a quick-fix recipe full of vitamins and fiber. Have it for lunch or dinner, especially when you are out of time, or do not have the inclination to spend more than 15 minutes in the kitchen.

Ingredients:

1 zucchini washed and sliced

1 can of mashed salmon

1/3 bunch of chopped dill

Juice of 1 freshly squeezed lemon

Sea salt or Himalayan Salt

2 tbsp olive oil


Preparation:

1. Beat the olive oil, salt, and lemon juice together into a vinaigrette.

2. Mix the zucchini, salmon, and dill.

3. Pour the vinaigrette over the zucchini mixture, and mix.

4. Your salad is ready to serve.

## *Blueberry Power Smoothie*

This is a fiber-rich, power-packed smoothie, full of vitamins and minerals. It can relieve constipation and give you an energy boost. This is also a good option to include in your detox diet.

Ingredients:

1 cup pineapple cut into small pieces

1 cup watermelon pieces

½ cup chopped baby spinach

½ a green apple, peeled and diced

2 cups fresh or frozen blueberries

2 quarts coconut water

Preparation:

Throw in all the ingredients into a blender, and blend in to a delicious smoothie.

## Apple and Celery Smoothie

This is a nutritious recipe packed with iron and healthy calories. It also works beautifully in flushing out toxins from your body.

Ingredients:

1 green apple cut into small pieces without peeling

1 stalk of celery

1 tablespoon of flaxseeds

1 pinch of cinnamon powder

1/3 cup of cilantro or parsley

1 cup kale

Juice of 1 whole freshly squeezed lemon

Preparation:

Add all the ingredients to a blender and blend into a healthy and delicious smoothie.

## Exercise

Exercise helps regulate the thyroid hormones, and stimulates your brain to secrete endorphins or feel-good hormones such as serotonin. Serotonin is important to counter depression, fatigue, and sleep disturbances. It can also help increase your appetite.

Hypothyroidism can make you gain almost 20 pounds of weight. It also makes you feel tired and fatigued all the time. Including at least 45 minutes to an hour of exercise routines in your daily schedule can help you lose weight, feel refreshed, happy, and less tired all the time.

However, hypothyroidism is often associated with adrenal fatigue, heart problems, and bone calcium loss due to thyroxine treatment. Thus, select your preferred form of exercise carefully. Do not over-exert yourself as this can further damage your thyroid functions. Avoid strenuous exercises if you have any underlying disorders. Try to exercise in the open as much as possible so that you benefit from fresh air and sunlight. Always begin gradually with 10 - 15 minute workout sessions, slowly increasing them to one-hour sessions. As your endurance or stamina increases, you can increase your exercise routines.

## Walking and jogging

Get yourself with a pair of running shoes, and you are ready to go. This is the easiest and cheapest form of exercise. You will certainly benefit from walking for one hour or jogging for 30 - 45 minutes daily or at least three to four times a week. Brisk walking at a speed that cover one km in seven - 10 minutes is ideal. You can gradually increase your exercise from walking to jogging and running, as your endurance increases.

## Mild Aerobics and Pilates

These are low intensity exercise forms, ideal for hypothyroidism, adrenal fatigue, and heart problems. These exercises bring about weight loss slowly by improving your metabolism. Aerobics is a set of coordinated dance moves involving stretching and strengthening exercises, while Pilates works on your back and spine.

## Cycling and swimming

If you are the sporty type, these exercises are for you. Do them in moderation, and do not strain yourself. Cycling works on the lower body muscles, bringing about weight loss, while swimming exercises the entire body against the forces of water. These are open-air exercises that will also help refresh you.

If your fatigue or tiredness increases, or you experience pain with exercise, stop whatever it is you are doing. Such physical stress will only make your thyroid gland more underactive. Instead, you can try yoga and meditation techniques. Yoga helps regulate metabolism, body functions in general, and has a calming effect. It also promotes weight loss by improving your metabolism. You can also practice yoga and meditation at the end of your workout.

## Yoga and Meditation

Yoga is an ancient Indian form or prayer and meditation. It harmonizes the energy forces in your body with those in the atmosphere, and soothes your mind and body.

Yoga, with its mind-body techniques, can regularize your hormones, reduce stress, and counter fatigue by increasing your energy levels. This spiritual healing art enhances your blood circulation and body movements. The various yoga asanas or exercises stretch your spine, removing the energy blocks along it. Yoga also improves detoxification by increasing blood circulation and metabolic activity. You can try some of the following meditation techniques and asanas.

However, if you experience pain while performing any of these exercises discontinue them. If possible, consult a trained or certified yoga instructor to master these techniques perfectly.

- **Surya namaskar or sun salutation:** Perform this pose first thing in the morning. Stand erect, with your feet together, hands pressed along your sides, keeping your palms open. Inhale and simultaneously sweep your hands upwards to join your palms above your head. Now exhale and bend forwards from your waist and hold your shins. Inhale again and move your torso upwards while you hold your shins to stretch your spine. Now exhale and bend forwards. Move back to an erect posture, join your hands in prayer, and take a deep breath. Once you have mastered this sequence do it five to six times daily.

- **Utrasana or camel pose:** This sequence works on the upper body, expands the lungs, and improves breathing. It also improves the blood circulation in the torso, and thus it can have positive effects on your thyroid gland. Kneel down so that you keep your upper body erect. Rest your palms on your hips and stretch backwards. You can try to touch your heels slowly, as your flexibility improves.

- These poses are effective only when performed skillfully. However, if you are unable to perform them, you can do simple breathing exercises and meditation. Simple meditation is easy to perform, and it effectively soothes the mind. It is a useful stress buster.

- **Simple meditation technique:** Sit erect on a chair or lie down on your bed. Close your eyes and concentrate on your breathing. When you feel your mind is clear of unpleasant or any thoughts, start thinking about happy thoughts, incidences, or places. Little by little, you will feel yourself relax and you will calm down.

- Another meditation technique recommended for hypothyroidism is to close your eyes and imagine a blue light entering your thyroid. This is known as color therapy, and the color blue is healing and associated with the throat chakra.

# Herbs and Alternative or Holistic Therapies to Heal Hypothyroidism

Herbs and holistic remedies are effective options to treat hypothyroidism and its accompanying symptoms. These therapies are often more successful in treating hypothyroidism as compared to conventional hormone replacement therapy.

Moreover, the upside to these remedies is that they seldom have any side effects. On the contrary, they can also ease the various side effects or conventional therapy. They also do not have any toxic effects on your body and can be safely taken along with western medicines.

## *Home remedies for hypothyroidism*

These remedies are known to improve general health and well-being, in addition to producing beneficial effects on your thyroid. You also need not look far for them. Most of these remedies are easily available in your kitchen or in the supermarkets.

*Ginger:* Ginger root is rich in potassium, zinc, and magnesium. Ginger also has powerful anti-inflammatory properties. It can improve your thyroid functions. You can add few pieces of dried or fresh ginger to your food or prepare ginger teas to gain from its health benefits. Ginger tea is prepared by boiling five to six pieces of ginger root fresh or dry, in a covered pot of water for five to seven minutes. Strain this infusion and add a teaspoon of honey to it.

*Kale, black walnuts, and Irish moss:* These herbs are rich in iodine. They improve metabolism, increase blood circulation, and enhance thyroid activity. You prepare herbal teas using these herbs. The method of preparation is similar to the ginger tea.

## Homeopathic remedies

Homeopathy is a relatively recent therapy among alternative cures. This effective holistic therapy cures the body and mind together, with little or no side effects.

It takes into consideration the entire disease picture including the underlying causative factors, unlike conventional medicines, which only give symptomatic relief making homeopathy a the perfect choice of treatment for hypothyroidism. It can successfully relieve your symptoms, stimulate your thyroid to work, and improve your metabolism. It also helps counter the side effects of thyroxine.

Here are some remedies out of the vast homeopathic pharmacopoeia that you can use to gain relief from your hypothyroid symptoms. However, for a complete and individualized cure, visit a registered homeopathic physician.

*Calcarea carbonicum:* This is one of the best and most commonly indicated homeopathic remedy for hypothyroidism. It is usually indicated for hypothyroidism in fat, obese, and flabby individuals.

Excess sweating, craving for boiled eggs, indigestion on eating fats, constipation, lethargy, and decreased metabolic rate and assimilation due to hypothyroidism, are effectively treated with calcarea carbonicum. It also works well in women experiencing excessive menstrual bleeding due to hypothyroidism. Calcarea carbonicum can also increase the calcium absorption in your body.

*Natrum muriaticum:* This remedy is prepared from common salt or natrum. Excessive craving for salt in food, depression with brooding, enlarged thyroid gland, constipation, and a decreased metabolic rate are indications of natrum muriaticum.

*Graphites:* This remedy is indicated for people with hyperthyroidism, who are obese, take on cold easily, suffer from chronic constipation characterized by hard lumpy motions, are depressed with a tendency to weep on listening to music, and are timid. It effectively relieves the symptoms of hypothyroidism in such individuals.

You can also take homeopathic remedies for common illnesses such as indigestion, especially as conventional drugs for such ailments cannot be taken along with your thyroid pill.

You can use remedies such as nux vomica, arsenic, lycopodium, and natrum carbonicum for indigestion instead of antacids.

# Quick Action Steps to Help Heal Your Hypothyroidism

This chapter briefly puts all the above information together in a nutshell. These quick action steps are meant to help you integrate the natural healing techniques explained in this book, in your daily schedule. Although, all of this information may seem a lot to process at one time, it is quite easy to practice. You can heal yourself and take control of your thyroid successfully, with the following daily schedule:

- Sleep for at least 8-10 hours daily.

- Wake up, brush, have your thyroid pill, and do the suryanamaskar or sun salutation explained in the chapter on yoga.

- Have a wholesome and nutritious breakfast, preferably prepared from organic food items. You can have one of the smoothies mentioned above to kick start your day.

- Exercise for 45 minutes to one-hour daily or at least three days a week. You can perform a workout of your choice. Exercise will refresh you, burn calories, and keep you full of vigor through the day. Have plenty of fluids, water, and fresh juices to keep yourself hydrated and boost your metabolism during your workout session.

- Have a light snack of low-fat yoghurt, a fruit salad, or buttermilk or milk, and muesli after your workout to regain your energy. Apples and pears are bulky fruits that can help kill your hunger pangs. Sprinkle a spoonful of flaxseeds over your snack.

- Keep your workplace or home well ventilated and well lit in the mornings and early afternoons. You can also perform light stretching exercises and meditation technique during the day to reduce drowsiness.

- Have a wholesome, nutritious, and organic lunch cooked in coconut or olive oil.

- Take a power nap in the early afternoon ½ hour after your lunchtime, for 30-60 minutes.

- In the late afternoon, have a green tea or one of the herbal teas mentioned here. Avoid caffeine in the form or coffee or tea. You can also have a small snack of berries, nuts, seeds, and fruits with your green tea.

- Have an early light dinner, cooked using organic foods and olive or coconut oil. Have your dinner at least 2 hours before your bedtime. Sleeping immediately after your meals can considerably decrease your metabolism.

- Listen to some soothing music or do some light reading before your bedtime. Have a warm bath, or massage your head with some brahmi, sesame, or coconut oil to unwind, especially if you have had a stressful day.

- Avoid watching television or using your computer or iPad at this time. Also, avoid working late.

- In general, avoid eating goitrogenic foods, processed foods, and carbohydrates. Have more proteins, vitamins, and minerals. Have more of iodine rich seafood.

- Use home remedies and herbs for common illnesses. Try using homeopathic remedies for your hypothyroid symptoms too. Your requirement of the thyroid pill may gradually reduce with homeopathy.

- Go for your health check-ups and thyroid tests regularly. Do not stop or change the dose of your thyroid pills without consulting your doctor.

# Conclusion

I hope this book was able to help you stabilize your thyroid hormones and improve the quality of your life.

If you have successfully gotten rid of a few faulty habits, and initiated a positive change in yourself, I am happy to have helped in the process. The guidelines presented in this book, will certainly improve your thyroid functions, and give you the much-needed relief you are after.

The next step is to motivate yourself to continue living a healthy and fulfilling lifestyle.

Thank you and good luck!

*Christine Weil*

# Check out the other books in the Natural Health & Natural Cures Series

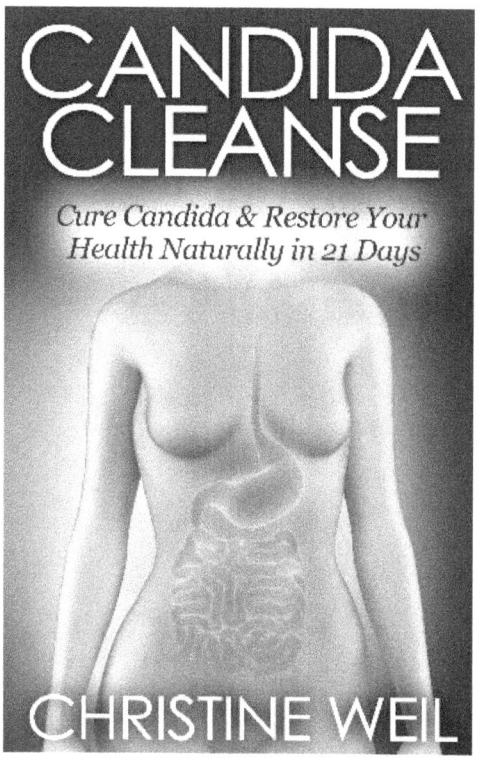

http://www.amazon.com/dp/B00IIRQH9K

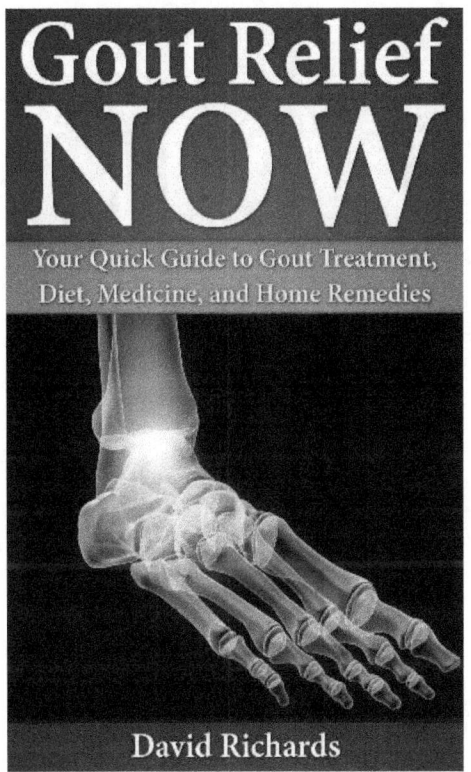

http://www.amazon.com/dp/B00HHGRBBQ

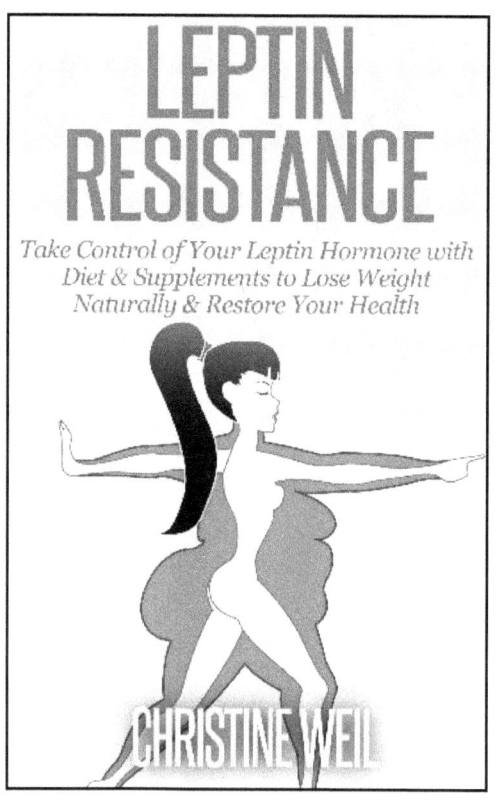

http://www.amazon.com/dp/B00J8UNBWW

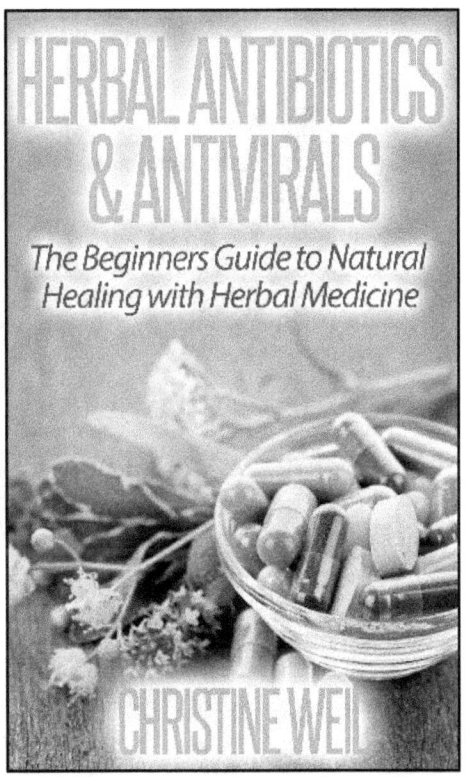

https://www.amazon.com/dp/B00J2F1QDO

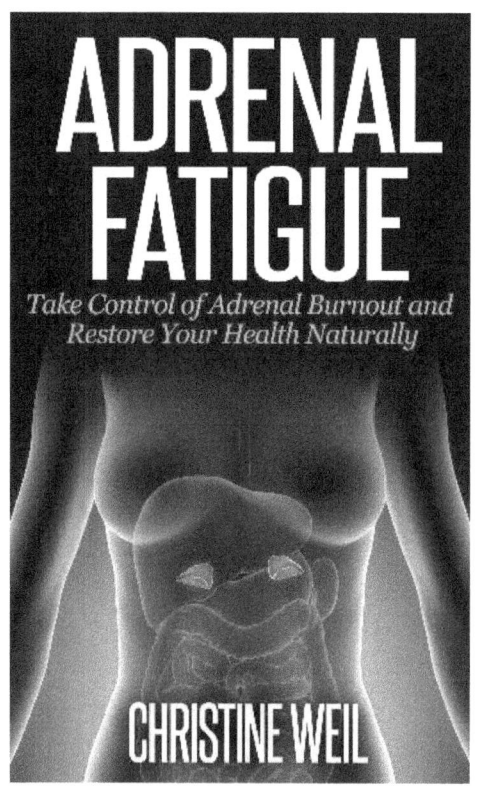

http://www.amazon.com/dp/B00J8SHS6E

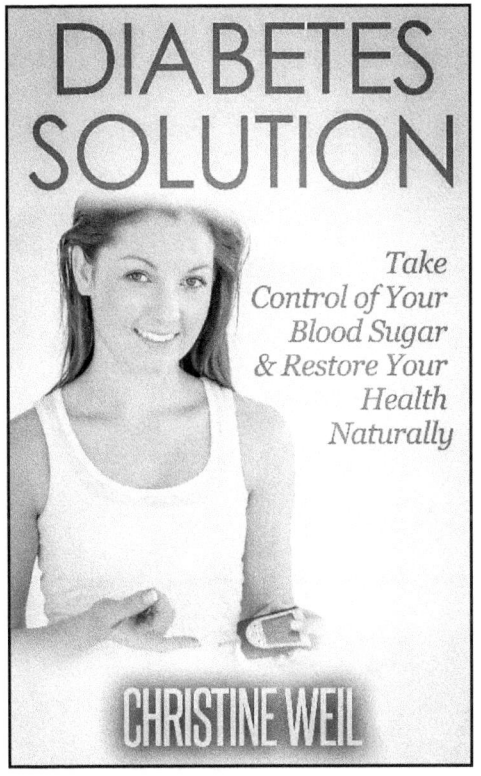

http://www.amazon.com/dp/B00KCAAKOO

www.ingramcontent.com/pod-product-compliance
Lightning Source LLC
Chambersburg PA
CBHW071626170526
45166CB00003B/1215